How to

Maintain & Keep

Happy Relationship

Building bond that lasts

Author bio

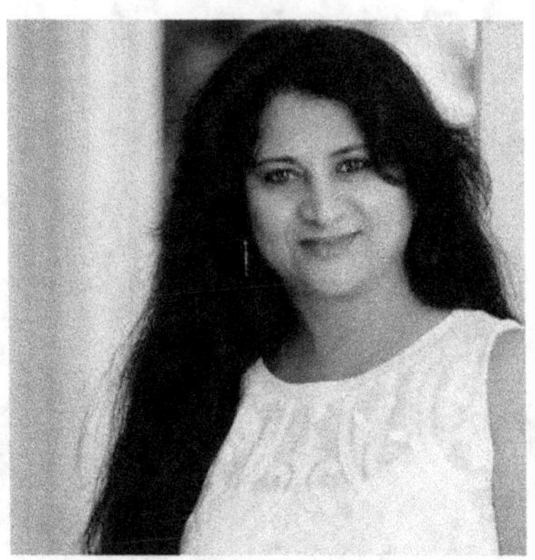

Dr. Vandana Bhalla earned her doctoral degree in Holistic Life Coaching from California, USA. With over two decades of dedicated practice in the fields of Holistic Health and personal development, she is a seasoned professional in her craft. Driven by her passion for empowering individuals, she shares her extensive knowledge and experience in self-care and holistic living.

Dr. Bhalla is deeply committed to assisting people in their journey toward achieving their aspirations and leading more meaningful lives. If you are someone who values health, happiness, and wellness, she invites you to join her newsletter and wellness community at https://dr-vandana.com

A HEALTHY RELATIONSHIP

Doesn't drag you down. It inspires you to be better

— Mandy Hale

TABLE OF CONTENT

INTRODUCTION

Relationships are like gardens; they require care, attention, and patience to flourish. In an era marked by fast-paced lives and ever-evolving dynamics, the art of building a healthy, lasting relationship can sometimes seem elusive. Yet, the quest for meaningful and enduring connections remains one of the most fundamental pursuits of human life. Whether you're just beginning a new relationship or seeking to rekindle the spark in an existing one, the principles that underpin lasting love are timeless.

Picture a relationship as a grand tapestry woven together with threads of communication, trust, quality time, empathy, conflict resolution, and individual growth. Each thread, when carefully tended to, strengthens the fabric of your connection, creating a bond that can withstand the tests of time and adversity. In this journey, we will look into the essential elements that compose the tapestry of a healthy relationship, unveiling the secrets to building a love that not only endures but also thrives.

From the importance of effective communication in fostering understanding to the bedrock of trust and transparency upon which lasting relationships are built, we will explain the intricacies of nurturing love. We will learn how to prioritize quality time, create meaningful rituals, and offer unwavering emotional support. Conflict, an inevitable part of any relationship, will be transformed from a potential source of strife into an opportunity for growth and resolution. And, in the midst of it all, we will discover the delicate balance between nurturing the partnership and nurturing individual identities.

Join us on this enlightening journey as we embark on the path to sustaining and enriching the love we share with our partners. Whether you are in a budding romance, a decades-long partnership, or simply seeking wisdom for future connections, the insights within these pages will illuminate the way forward. Let us embark on this exploration of the art of building a healthy relationship that stands the test of time, where love is not just an emotion but a lifelong commitment to growth, understanding, and shared joy

CHAPTER ONE: EFFECTIVE COMMUNICATION

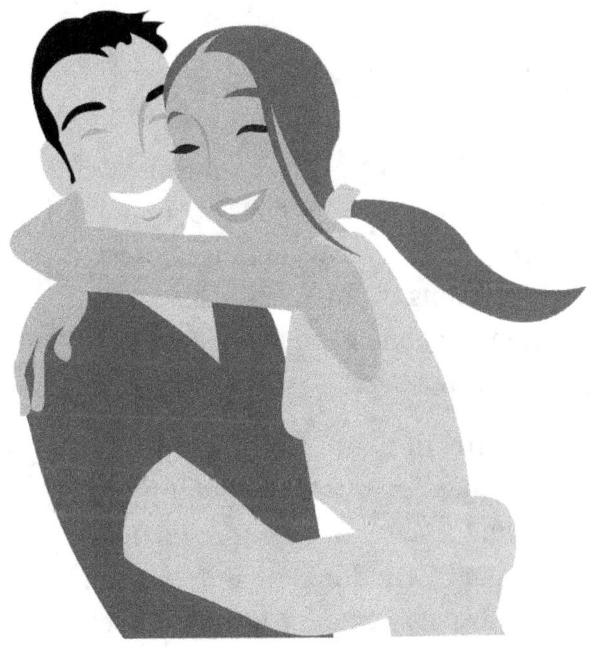

Effective communication is the cornerstone of maintaining and nurturing a healthy, lasting relationship. It's the bridge that connects two individuals, allowing them to understand, support, and love each other more deeply. In this exploration of communication within relationships, we'll go into various facets of human touch, both physical and emotional, and how they contribute to building and sustaining a strong bond.

Physical Attraction:

This is a powerful means of communication that goes beyond words. It encompasses a wide range of expressions, from a gentle caress to a warm hug, and each touch conveys a unique message:

* **Affection and Connection:** This is a way to express affection, intimacy, and a sense of belonging. Holding hands, cuddling, or simply sitting close can create a profound feeling of connection.

* **Comfort and Support:** In times of distress or sadness, a comforting touch on the shoulder or a reassuring

hug can convey support and empathy when words may fall short.

* **Passion and Desire:** Intimacy plays a vital role in romantic relationships, serving as a way to express desire, passion, and love. It fosters a deep emotional connection and strengthens the romantic bond.

* **Apology and Reconciliation:** A heartfelt apology can be amplified by a sincerity. It communicates remorse and the desire to mend any hurt feelings.

* **Non-Verbal Communication:** This often complements verbal communication. A loving pat on the back or a gentle squeeze of the hand can affirm agreement, understanding, or solidarity.

Emotional Attraction:

Communication within a healthy relationship extends beyond physical touch; it also involves emotional attraction:

* **Empathy and Understanding:** This is about acknowledging your partner's feelings on a profound level. It means being emotionally available, actively listening, and offering understanding and validation.

* **Vulnerability and Trust:** Sharing your own emotions and vulnerabilities builds trust and intimacy. When you open up to your partner, it encourages them to do the same.

* **Validation and Appreciation:** Expressing appreciation for your partner's thoughts, efforts, and feelings is a form of emotional attraction. It validates their importance within the relationship

Verbal Communication:

While the above discussed are potent means of communication, verbal communication remains essential in maintaining a healthy relationship:

* **Open and Honest Dialogue:** Encourage open and honest conversations. Share your thoughts, concerns, and aspirations, and invite your partner to do the same. This helps build trust and transparency.

* **Active Listening:** Effective communication is a two-way street. Actively listen when your partner speaks, and seek to understand their perspective before responding. Show that you value their thoughts and feelings.

* **Conflict Resolution:** Conflicts are inevitable in any relationship. Healthy communication involves addressing issues respectfully,

finding compromise, and working together to resolve disagreements.

❖ **Words of Affection:** Don't underestimate the power of words to express love and appreciation. Regularly tell your partner how much they mean to you and why you cherish them.

In conclusion, effective communication in a healthy relationship involves a harmonious blend of physical attraction, emotional attraction, and verbal communication. It's a dynamic process that requires ongoing effort, patience, and understanding. When partners learn to communicate effectively through touch and words, they create a deep, lasting connection that can weather life's challenges and grow stronger with time.

Communication

Goals

Goals ...

Steps For Achieving

Step 1.

____

____

____

Step 2.

____

____

____

Step 3.

____

____

____

CHAPTER TWO: TRUST AND TRANSPARENCY

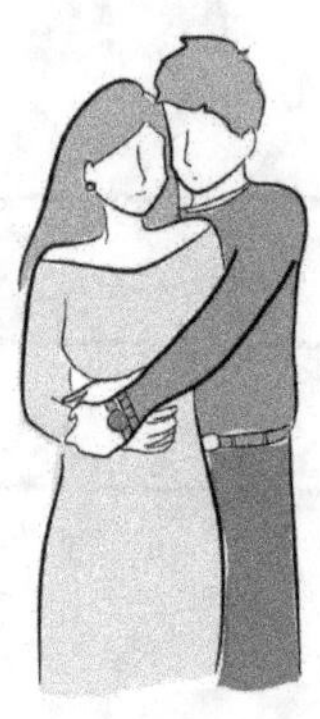

Trust and transparency are the bedrock of a healthy, enduring relationship. They are like the nourishing soil in which the seeds of love and connection can flourish. In this exploration of trust and transparency, we will explain the profound ways we can foster and reinforce these vital elements within a relationship.

Building Trust through Human Touch

Human touch is a visceral, primal means of building trust. It conveys vulnerability, intimacy, and authenticity:

❖ **Physical Presence:** Simply being physically present with your partner can be a powerful trust-builder. Holding hands, cuddling, or sharing an embrace can reassure your partner of your commitment and presence in their life.

❖ **Consistency:** Regular, affectionate touch communicates consistency and reliability. When your partner knows they can count on your physical affection, it strengthens their trust in the relationship.

❖ **Physical Intimacy:** In romantic relationships, physical intimacy fosters trust by creating a unique bond between partners. It's a vulnerable act that says, "I trust you with my body and my heart."

❖ Comfort in Vulnerability: Trust is also about being able to be vulnerable with your partner. Human touch can offer comfort and reassurance during times of vulnerability, reinforcing the belief that your partner is a safe haven.

Fostering Transparency

Transparency within a relationship involves open, honest, and authentic communication. This plays a significant role in supporting this:

- ❖ **Physical Comfort:** When you or your partner shares your thoughts and feelings, offering physical comfort through, it can make it easier to open up. A reassuring hand on the shoulder or a warm hug can provide emotional safety.

- ❖ **Emotional Attraction:** Emotional attraction involves conveying your emotions through physical gestures. For instance, a passionate kiss can convey love and desire, while a gentle touch can express tenderness and care.

- ❖ **Affirming Honesty:** When discussing sensitive topics or making

  important decisions, this can affirm your commitment to honesty. Holding your partner's hand as you share difficult truths shows that you are dedicated to transparency in the relationship.

❖ **Celebrating Authenticity:**
Transparency also means celebrating
each other's true selves. When you
touch your partner with genuine
affection, you validate their
authenticity and encourage them to
be themselves.

Rebuilding Trust and Reestablishing Transparency

In situations where trust has been
compromised or transparency has
wavered, human touch can play a vital
role in the healing process:

❖ **Forgiveness and Reassurance:**
When working through trust issues,
physical touch can be a way to
express forgiveness and reassure
your partner of your commitment to
rebuilding the relationship.

❖ **Reconnecting:** After a period of emotional distance, reconnecting through touch can be a powerful means of reestablishing trust and transparency.

❖ **Physical Boundaries:** Respect each other's physical boundaries as an essential aspect of trust and transparency. Ensure that any physical touch is consensual and comfortable for both partners.

In conclusion, human touch is not just a physical act; it is a profound means of conveying trust, transparency, and emotional authenticity within a relationship. When used thoughtfully and respectfully, touch can reinforce the foundation of trust and nurture the authenticity required for a healthy and enduring partnership.

Trust & Transparency Goals

Goals …

Steps For Achieving

Step 1.

____

____

____

Step 2.

____

____

____

Step 3.

____

____

____

CHAPTER THREE: QUALITY TIME TOGETHER

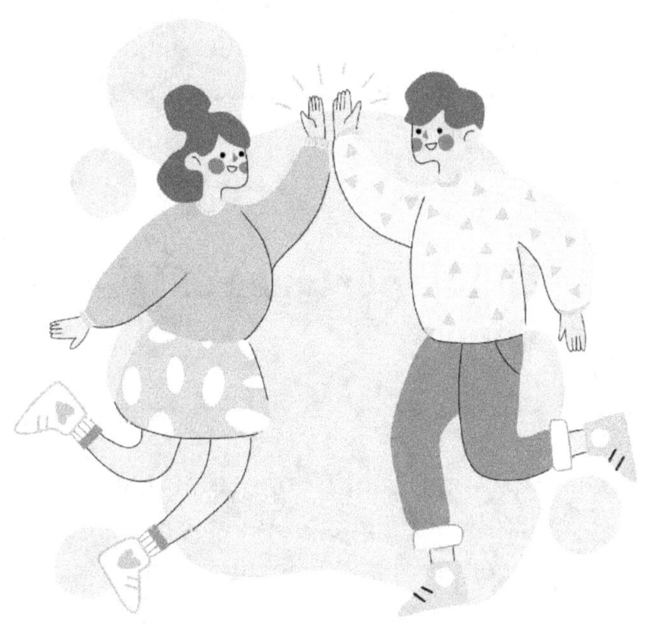

In the fast-paced world we live in, where schedules are often hectic and distractions are abundant, the concept of quality time together takes on paramount importance in maintaining and nurturing a healthy, lasting relationship. Quality time isn't merely about being physically present; it's about engaging in meaningful, fulfilling activities that strengthen the bond between partners. In this exploration of quality time, we'll make known why it matters and how to ensure it remains a cornerstone of your relationship.

The Importance of Quality Time

❖ **Emotional Connection:** Quality time together cultivates a profound emotional connection. It allows partners to share experiences, thoughts, and feelings, deepening their understanding of one another.

❖ **Rekindling Romance:** In romantic relationships, dedicating quality time helps rekindle the flames of passion and desire. It provides opportunities for intimacy and physical closeness, fostering a sense of romance.

- ❖ **Stress Relief:** Spending quality time with your partner can serve as a potent stress reliever. It offers a break from the demands of daily life and provides a safe space for relaxation and rejuvenation.

- ❖ **Building Memories:** Quality time leads to the creation of cherished memories. These shared experiences become the foundation of your unique history together, reinforcing your sense of togetherness.

Tips for Maintaining Quality Time

- ❖ **Prioritize Time Management:** Allocate time in your schedule for your relationship. Just as you schedule work meetings or appointments, make sure you have dedicated time for your partner.

❖ **Unplug and Disconnect:** To truly engage in quality time, it's essential to disconnect from electronic devices and distractions. This allows you to be fully present with your partner.

❖ **Plan Special Activities:** Consider planning activities that both you and your partner enjoy. It could be anything from cooking a meal together, taking a nature walk, or pursuing a shared hobby.

❖ **Quality Over Quantity:** Quality time doesn't have to be extensive; it just needs to be meaningful. If the time being dedicated to one's partner isn't used for something meaningful, that's not encouraging. Even short, focused periods of connection can have a significant impact.

- ❖ **Communication:** Communicate with your partner about your expectations and desires regarding quality time. Understand what activities resonate with them and what makes them feel most connected.

- ❖ **Surprise Gestures:** Surprise your partner with unexpected acts of love and attention. It could be as simple as leaving a love note or planning a spontaneous date night.

- ❖ **Respect Each Other's Interests:** While shared activities are essential, also respect each other's individual interests. Encourage your partner to pursue their passions, even if they differ from yours.

Overcoming Challenges:

- ❖ **Balancing Responsibilities:** Finding time for quality moments can be challenging when balancing work, family, and other responsibilities. It requires thoughtful scheduling and prioritization.

❖ **Long-Distance Relationships:** In long-distance relationships, quality time often involves virtual communication. Consistency and creativity in maintaining connections are crucial.

❖ **Relationship Ruts:** Over time, relationships may fall into routines. To overcome this, explore new activities, revisit old hobbies, or embark on adventures together to inject excitement into your quality time.

In conclusion, quality time is not just a luxury; it's a necessity for maintaining a healthy and enduring relationship. By investing in meaningful experiences and genuine connection, partners can strengthen their emotional bonds, reignite their passion, and create a

love that stands the test of time. Quality
time is the key to nurturing a relationship
that continues to thrive, even in the
busiest of lives.

Quality Time
Goals

Goals ...

Steps For Achieving

Step 1.

Step 2.

Step 3.

CHAPTER FOUR: EMOTIONAL SUPPORT AND EMPATHY

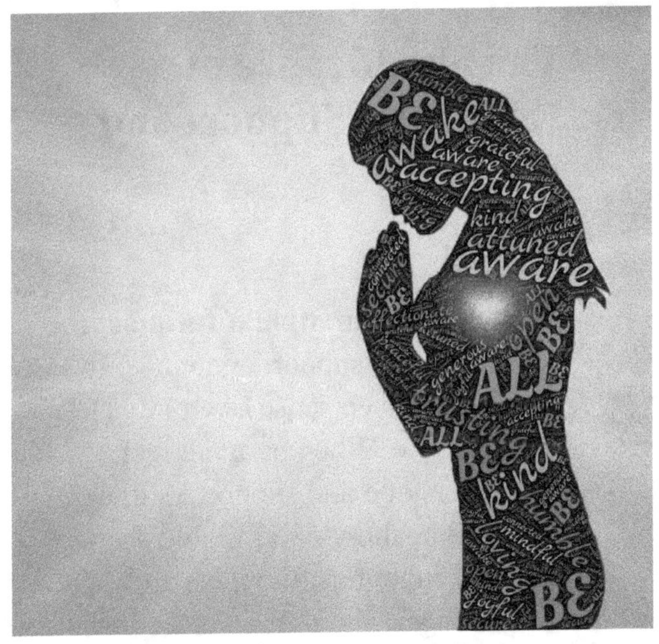

Emotional support and empathy
are the lifeblood of a thriving, lasting

relationship. These qualities create a safe and nurturing environment in which partners can express themselves, lean on each other during challenging times, and celebrate each other's joys. In this comprehensive exploration, we will look into the significance of emotional support and empathy, and how they can be cultivated to maintain and keep a healthy relationship.

The Significance of Emotional Support and Empathy

- ❖ **Creating Emotional Intimacy:** Emotional support and empathy foster a deep sense of emotional intimacy. When partners feel understood and supported, they become more comfortable sharing their innermost thoughts and feelings.

- ❖ **Strengthening Trust:** Trust is the foundation of any healthy relationship, and emotional support plays a crucial role in building and maintaining that trust. When you consistently offer support, your partner learns they can rely on you during both good and bad times.

❖ **Conflict Resolution:** Empathy is essential in resolving conflicts. It allows you to see things from your partner's perspective, facilitating compromise and understanding during disagreements.

❖ **Boosting Resilience:** Emotional support helps both partners cope with life's challenges. When you know your partner is there for you, it becomes easier to face adversity with resilience and courage.

Cultivating Emotional Support and Empathy

❖ **Active Listening:** Practice active listening when your partner is sharing their thoughts and feelings. Give them your full attention, ask open-ended questions to understand better, and avoid interrupting.

❖ **Validate Feelings:** Show empathy by acknowledging your partner's emotions. Say things like, "I understand how you must be feeling" or "It's okay to feel this way." Validation makes your partner feel heard and understood.

❖ **Be Present:** Being emotionally present means setting aside distractions and truly engaging with your partner. Whether in joyful moments or during difficult times, your presence communicates your support.

❖ **Offer Comfort:** In times of distress, offer emotional comfort. This can be through physical, comforting words, or simply being there as a source of solace.

- ❖ **Share Your Own Feelings:** Emotional support is a two-way street. Don't hesitate to share your own feelings and vulnerabilities with your partner. This openness encourages them to reciprocate.

- ❖ **Practice Empathy:** Put yourself in your partner's shoes. Try to understand their perspective and emotions, even if you don't fully agree or comprehend. Empathy is about showing that you care about their feelings.

Challenges in Offering Support and Empathy

- ❖ **Burnout:** It's essential to balance emotional support with self-care.

Constantly giving without taking time for yourself can lead to burnout. Make sure to communicate your own needs as well.

❖ **Misunderstandings:** Sometimes, despite your best efforts, you may misunderstand your partner's emotions. In such cases, open communication is key. Encourage your partner to clarify their feelings and concerns.

❖ **Avoiding Fixing:** It's important to understand that emotional support doesn't always mean offering solutions. Sometimes, your partner may simply need someone to listen and validate their feelings without trying to fix the problem.

In conclusion, emotional support and empathy are the threads that weave the fabric of a strong, healthy relationship. When partners consistently provide these essential qualities, they create a haven of trust, understanding, and comfort. Through the highs and lows of life, emotional support and empathy serve as the glue that keeps a relationship resilient, nurturing, and enduring.

Emotional Support-
Goals

____

____

____

____

____

____

____

____

____

____

____

Goals …

Steps For Achieving

Step 1.

____

____

____

Step 2.

____

____

____

Step 3.

____

____

____

CHAPTER FIVE: CONFLICT RESOLUTION

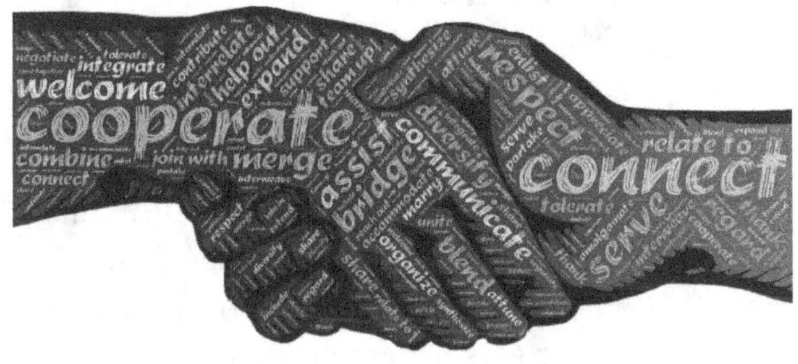

Conflict is a natural and inevitable part of any relationship. It's not the presence of conflict that jeopardizes a relationship; rather, it's how conflicts are managed and resolved. Effective conflict resolution is a cornerstone of maintaining a healthy, lasting relationship. In this comprehensive exploration, we'll simplify the significance of conflict resolution and provide guidance on how to navigate turbulent waters while strengthening your connection.

The Significance of Conflict Resolution:

* **Understanding Differences:** Conflict often arises from differences in values, needs, or perspectives. Effectively resolving conflicts helps partners better understand each other, leading to a deeper connection.

* **Strengthening Communication:** Healthy conflict resolution encourages open and honest communication. It creates a safe space for partners to express their thoughts and feelings without fear of judgment.

❖ **Preventing Resentment:**
Unresolved conflicts can fester and lead to resentment. Regularly addressing issues and finding solutions prevents these negative emotions from eroding the relationship.

❖ **Fostering Growth:** Conflict can be an opportunity for personal and relational growth. It challenges individuals to adapt, compromise, and find common ground.

Effective Conflict Resolution Strategies:

❖ **Stay Calm:** In the heat of an argument, emotions can run high. Try to stay calm and composed, and encourage your partner to do the same. Take breaks if needed to cool off before continuing the discussion.

❖ **Active Listening:** Truly hear your partner's perspective. Practice active listening by giving them your full attention and seeking to understand their point of view before responding.

❖ **Use "I" Statements:** Instead of blaming or accusing, use "I" statements to express your feelings and needs. For example, say, "I feel hurt when..." rather than "You always…"

❖ **Seek Compromise:** Conflict resolution often involves finding a middle ground. Be willing to compromise and collaborate on solutions that work for both partners.

❖ **Choose Your Battles:** Not every issue requires a full-blown argument. Consider whether the conflict is worth the emotional energy and, if not, let it go.

❖ **Stay Respectful:** Maintain respect for your partner even during disagreements. Avoid name-calling, insults, or hurtful language.

❖ **Find Common Goals:** Remind yourselves of your shared goals and values. This can help put the conflict in perspective and motivate you to work through it together.

Challenges in Conflict Resolution:

❖ **Emotional Intensity:** Strong emotions can cloud judgment and hinder effective resolution. It's important to recognize when emotions are escalating and take steps to calm down before continuing the discussion.

- ❖ **Unresolved Past Issues:** Sometimes, conflicts stem from unresolved issues from the past. It's essential to address these underlying concerns and not let them fester.

- ❖ **Different Conflict Styles:** Partners may have different approaches to conflict. Some may prefer to discuss issues immediately, while others may need time to process. Finding a balance in conflict styles is key.

- ❖ **External Stressors:** External stressors like work, finances, or health can exacerbate conflicts. In such cases, it's important to acknowledge the impact of external factors on your relationship and work together to mitigate their effects.

In conclusion, conflict resolution is not about avoiding disagreements but about managing them constructively. By approaching conflicts with patience, respect, and a commitment to finding

solutions, partners can transform
moments of tension into opportunities
for growth and deeper connection. When
conflicts are addressed with care, a
healthy relationship becomes even
stronger, more resilient, and better
equipped to weather the challenges of
life together.

Conflict Resolution - Goals

Goals ...

Steps For Achieving

Step 1.

____

____

____

Step 2.

____

____

____

Step 3.

____

____

____

CHAPTER SIX: MAINTAINING INDIVIDUAL IDENTITIES

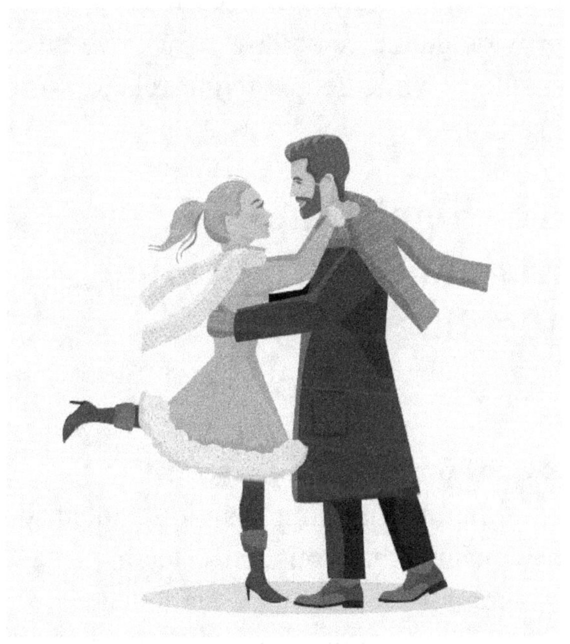

In the pursuit of a healthy and lasting relationship, one often hears about the importance of togetherness and unity. While these aspects are indeed crucial, it's equally vital to maintain individual identities within a partnership. This delicate balance between "we" and "me" is essential for nurturing a relationship that thrives and endures. In this comprehensive exploration, we'll delve into the significance of maintaining individual identities and provide guidance on how to achieve this harmony while keeping your relationship healthy.

The Significance of Maintaining Individual Identities:

❖ **Preserving Self-Esteem:** Maintaining your individual identity ensures that your self-esteem remains intact. It's a reminder that you are a unique, valuable person independent of the relationship.

❖ **Fostering Personal Growth:** A healthy relationship encourages

personal growth. When you pursue
your individual interests and
aspirations, you continue to evolve
and bring new experiences and
perspectives into the relationship.

❖ **Preventing Codependency:**
Codependency, where one partner
becomes overly reliant on the other,
can be detrimental to a relationship.
Maintaining individual identities
helps prevent this by ensuring both
partners have a sense of self and
independence.

❖ **Enriching the Relationship:** When
partners maintain their individual
identities, they have more to bring to
the relationship. Unique interests,
experiences, and skills can enhance
the partnership and keep it vibrant.

Strategies for Maintaining Individual Identities:

❖ **Pursue Personal Interests:** Continue to engage in activities and hobbies that are important to you. Dedicate time to your passions, whether it's a hobby, career pursuit, or personal goals.

❖ **Set Boundaries:** Establish clear boundaries to ensure you have personal space and time. Communicate your needs for solitude or time with friends and family, and respect your partner's boundaries as well.

❖ **Encourage Each Other:** Support each other's individual aspirations and personal growth. Encourage your partner to pursue their goals and be their biggest cheerleader.

- ❖ **Maintain Social Connections:** Don't neglect your social circle and friendships. Maintain relationships with friends and family outside of the partnership to stay connected to your support network.

- ❖ **Communication is Key:** Open communication is vital. Talk with your partner about your need for personal space and the importance of maintaining individual identities within the relationship.

- ❖ **Prioritize Self-Care:** Take care of your physical and mental health. Self-care is not selfish; it's a necessary component of maintaining your individual well-being.

Challenges in Maintaining Individual Identities:

- ❖ **Fear of Neglect:** Some individuals fear that pursuing their own interests will lead to neglecting the relationship. It's important to communicate with your partner and reassure them that personal growth benefits the partnership.

❖ **Balance in Time Management:** Balancing personal interests, work, and the relationship can be challenging. Effective time management and prioritization are key.

❖ **Respect for Differences:** Partners may have different needs when it comes to maintaining their individual identities. It's important to respect these differences and find a balance that works for both.

❖ **Overcoming Societal Expectations:** Societal norms often emphasize the idea of total togetherness in a relationship. Overcoming these expectations and recognizing the value of individuality can be a challenge.

In conclusion, maintaining individual identities within a relationship is not about distancing oneself from a partner but about nurturing personal growth, self-esteem, and independence. When both partners continue to evolve as individuals, they bring more richness and depth to the relationship. This balance between individuality and togetherness is the foundation of a healthy, thriving, and enduring partnership

Maintain Individual Identity -Goals

____

____

____

____

Goals ...

____

____

____

____

____

____

____

____

Steps For Achieving

Step 1.

____

Step 2.

____

____

____

Step 3.

____

____

____

CONCLUSION

In the journey we've undertaken through these pages, we've explored the intricate web of ingredients that form the tapestry of a healthy, lasting relationship. From effective communication and trust to quality time, emotional support, conflict resolution, and the preservation of individual identities, we've unveiled the secrets to nurturing a love that endures.

But beyond the practical advice and strategies, the essence of this book lies in the profound understanding that a healthy relationship is not an end goal but a continuous, evolving journey. It's a journey marked by growth, connection, understanding, and unwavering commitment.

As you read to the conclusion of this book, remember that the insights you've gained are not merely concepts to ponder; they are tools to be put into practice. They are the threads you weave into your relationship, creating a tapestry that reflects the uniqueness of your love story.

Who Will Benefit From This Book?

❖ **Couples at Every Stage:** Whether you're embarking on a new relationship, celebrating years of togetherness, or seeking to rekindle the spark, the principles shared here apply to couples at every stage of their journey.

❖ **Individuals Ready for Love:** For those seeking love or preparing for a new relationship, this book provides invaluable guidance on building a strong foundation and fostering healthy connections.

❖ **Counselors and Therapists:** Professionals in the field of relationship counseling and therapy will find this book to be a valuable resource to recommend to their clients. It offers practical insights to support clients in their relationship journeys.

- ❖ **Friends and Family:** Friends and family members looking to offer support and advice to their loved ones in relationships can benefit from the wisdom shared within these pages.

- ❖ **Self-Explorers:** Even if you're not currently in a relationship, this book offers valuable insights into self-awareness, emotional intelligence, and personal growth that can enrich your life in various ways.

Remember that the most enduring love stories are not without their challenges, but they are marked by the commitment to face those challenges together. The lessons you've gleaned from these pages can serve as a guiding light, helping you navigate the intricacies of love with wisdom, compassion, and resilience.

May your journey in love be a beautiful tapestry, woven with threads of understanding, trust, and enduring affection. As you move forward, may you find inspiration in the knowledge that the power to nurture lasting love lies within your hands and hearts.

***

Relationship Journal

____

____

Notes ...

Notes ...

Notes …

Congratulations!

Have Joyful, trusted and
long-lasting
relationships blessings